The

Metamorphosis Of Princess Kizziemae

Confessions of a Fat Girl

Beverly A. Rivers

PUBLISHING INFORMATION

ISBN: 978-1-105-40562-4 (Revision 1)

Published by Beverly A. Rivers

CAUTION

It is strongly recommended that you consult your physician for professional advice on weight loss or addictive behaviors. This book is solely for inspirational purposes.

CONTENTS

Making That Change

Appendix

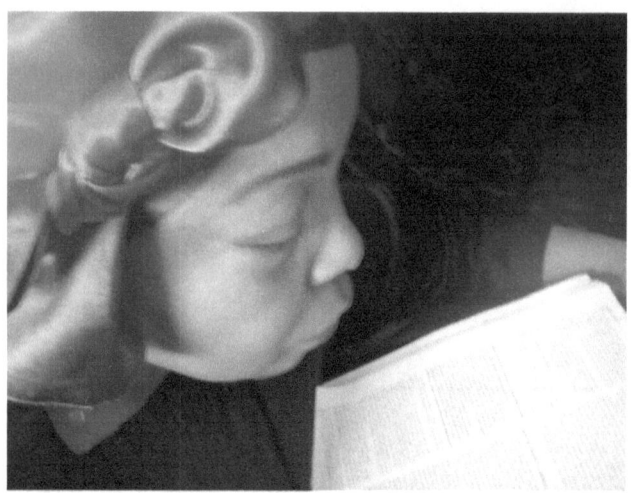

Forward

In July of 2010 I began a natural hair care journey. My initial plan was to grow my hair under wigs for a few months until I could learn how to style and wear it publicly. However, after arriving in Japan, the heat and humidity flushed me out of my wig and weave hair and I had to find other alternatives.

I learned many things by watching online video blogs of black women caring for and styling their natural hair. Many hours were invested in educating myself on techniques I didn't learn as I was growing up. Within a few months I decided to document my hair care journey.

Princess Kizziemae is my blogger name on Youtube. The name is inspired by a monologue I wrote in high school about a slave girl named Kizziemae who worked in the "big house for Mastuh John and Missy Ann". In the monologue Kizziemae asked her mama. "How cumz my hair is thick an' mossy likes cotton?" I performed that skit at age 16 in a high school variety show. It was a creative way of reaching out for answers about black womanhood. No one ever answered my many questions or offered any knowledge so I had to learn through life experience. Now, 36 years later I find myself looking for answers to the same questions. Kizziemae is the young girl in me who needs to process some things to be able to realize her full destiny in life.

As I began blogging, I took many weekly photos to document my progress. The pictures revealed that I had neglected not only my hair but my entire image. I began to see myself from the outside for the first time in a long time. It was truly eye opening to see hard evidence of this neglect in pictures that did not reflect how I see myself in my minds eye.

What began as a hair care journey quickly became a makeover journey. As of the completion of this book I have been on the journey for 15 months. Three months into the journey, I began to reflect on my life, asking myself some hard questions, and praying for understanding. How did I allow myself to fall apart like this? As I examined myself; body, soul, and spirit, many nuggets of understanding were revealed. As a result I am being transformed by the renewing of my mind.

Seeking out inspiration on the internet, I came across several two-year old weight loss journey blogs. There were people who successfully lost the weight, enjoyed it for a few months and soon gained it all back! Upon further search, I found the same persons doing another weight loss blog on a journey to lose the weight again. How exhausting!

With strong conviction, I decided to lose this weight for the very last time. Weight gain is no longer acceptable. My heart goes out to obese people like myself who struggle to attain and maintain the body size of their dreams. My goal is to share this journey and help as many others as I can. I'm here to prove to myself and others that we can overcome the barriers that stand in the way of a healthy body image and self esteem.

When I was young I didn't love and appreciate my body. Like most people, I compared myself to the media's example of beauty and labeled anything that didn't fit their mold… a flaw. My hair doesn't blow in the wind then gently descend to caress my shoulders like strands of silk. Thus my thin kinky, koily hair has been offensively labeled African slave hair by the people I grew up with. (Most of them are also Black/African American with the same hair texture.)

If I were to wear a tube top with no bra I'd be cited for indecent exposure. I have never worn a bikini on the beach or under my clothes either. It was never a comfortable garment for my body size. Nor have I ever worn a size 6 anything …not even a shoe …as an adult. My body size is a reflection of the people in my early childhood. We were all big!

In the southern states of Georgia and Florida where I spent my formative years, a woman with big hips, thighs, and curves who could cook was labeled a good catch. These women were considered healthy and sexy. Skinny women, on the other hand, were considered unattractive. However, when I moved to California, suddenly the whole definition changed. People on the West Coast were obsessed with being thin. The West Coast motto seemed to be; *the thinner the better*.

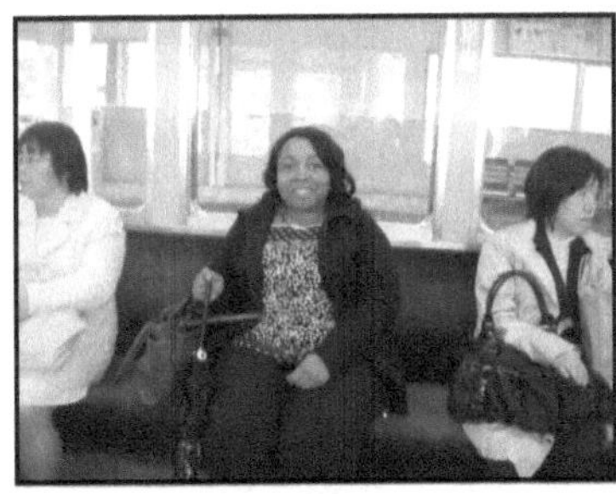

When I arrived in Japan, my size became even more noticeable. The average woman is about my height, but only about one half of my body size at that time. It is rare to see an obese Japanese person. Usually all of the oversized people here are foreigners.

In the photo above, I am sitting on a train in Japan beside one of few obese Japanese women. Ironically I noticed this as I was choosing photos for this book.

My Japanese friends are quick to use the word, FAT. They are the first to notice and comment on any weight loss or gain. Annoying? Yes! But overall it has blessed me and helped me to face facts.

Defining the ideal body has always been confusing. However, this I know for sure. Obesity is not healthy regardless of social acceptance or location. Even in the South, a woman lost beauty points if she allowed herself to become too big and sloppy. Soon folks would begin calling her a FAT gal. At the end of the day, no one else's opinion really matters except my own. I am not attractive to myself, and that's the catalyst for change.

There are many people who have attained the media's image of an ideal body with crash dieting, surgery, drugs, or other procedures. There have been many horror stories about the side effects and various health issues that followed. The ultimate healthy body has its foundation in good nutrition and exercise habits.

As a child, like many other little girls I wanted to be a ballerina, figure skater or a gymnast. But, I've given up wanting a dancer's body. Now I realize I have an athletic body. Naturally I have big muscles in my thighs and calves. I'm a bit on the stocky side. This was a key factor to consider when I set my target weight goal. The standard weight chart says that I should weigh between 104-137lbs depending upon my frame. I set my target weight at the high end, 135-140lbs. This was my pre-child bearing weight and is realistic and maintainable for my lifestyle. My goal is to be healthy, slim, look good in my clothes, feel attractive, and improve my self image. I want to love and dress my body in ways that make me feel and look beautiful. To begin moving in the right direction, something has to change. That something is inside of me.

Permanent change starts at the core of our being…our soul and spirit. When these two intangible parts of our being are healed, the body will follow. At the end of this book, you'll find questionnaires, worksheets, website listings and recipes that may be helpful. If you are reading this because you too are on a weight loss journey, I suggest that you take some time and answer the questions openly and honestly by writing your response in the space provided. Stop your world for a moment and take some time to evaluate where you are. Really dig deep.

Do your research. Surf the internet, read blogs, and watch video blogs online. Our bodies are similar but uniquely different. What works for me may not work with your body chemistry, lifestyle or family medical history. You've heard it many times before. Get a full physical exam to rule out any medical reasons that may cause you to be overweight.

I made my emotional health top priority for a while. As a result I woke up and recognized that I AM FAT but I have the power to change it. I'm on a journey for permanent change, so I'm not in a hurry.

This book is the first in a series of intermittent books to document and share what I'm learning along my journey. If I wait until I reach my goal, many of these experiences and revelations will no longer be fresh in my mind. In addition I will be enjoying new experiences in life and may no longer be motivated to rehash this topic.

Sharing as I go, will allow others to come along on this journey with me. Though everyone's body is different, my documented successes and failures may be an inspiration and give some help to others who have the same or similar struggles.

Confessions 1-2 are the wake up calls that motivated me to begin this journey. Confessions 3-7 are reflections on memories of old and new experiences that have shaped my thoughts about food and consequently shaped my body. Confessions 8-9 are the actions I took to lose the 50 pounds. Confession 10 is a dedication to an anonymous loved one who is morbidly obese. Finally, in the appendix at the end of the book, I share resources, recipes, and final thoughts to help you get your journey kick started.

Princess Kizziemae is beautiful, talented, and gifted yet she struggles to come out of her cocoon and be the lovely creature God intended from the beginning. You may find that you have some things in common with her. Princess Kizziemae must be healed so that Queen Beverly can emerge.

My readers will no doubt fall into one of three groups. Some are at a normal weight but are curious about what a fat girl might confess. Some are a bit overweight and bought this book hoping to pick up some weight loss tips. Others are obese and feel trapped in their bodies. Like me, they need encouragement and inspiration to believe that they can really lose the excess weight for good.

This book may be helpful in all of these areas. Along the way it will be entertaining, educational, and sometimes downright offensive. So be warned and get ready for a journey inside. . .

The Metamorphosis of Princess Kizziemae
Confessions of a FAT Girl.

CONFESSION ONE

Many wake up calls

In 2010 I was asked to do a three year teaching assignment in Japan. How exciting!! I've always dreamed of teaching music full time. I had no idea that accepting this assignment would cause me to take a long hard look at my health and the image I was projecting. I was asked to do a concert tour to promote a large music festival where at least ten thousand people were expected to attend. As a singer, songwriter, I thought this could be a tremendous blessing especially if I were asked to be one of the performers at such an event.

I was given this assignment on recommendation by my sponsor and sent out on tour a month before meeting the festival leaders. My hope to take that stage was very high. With expectation, I travelled to 20 locations in the hot Japanese humid summer sun to encourage people to attend. The attendees at these promotional concerts were constantly asking what day I would be performing at the festival.

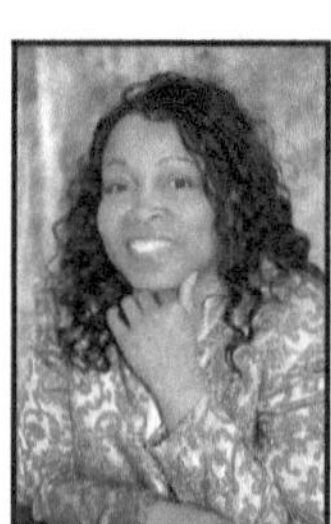

The promoters of the concert tour asked me to provide a publicity photo. Pictured to the left is the headshot I submitted. Beautiful, yes? This photo was taken in 2007 when I was about 30 pound lighter and wearing an attractive wavy weave hairdo.

Once I arrived in Japan, the weave had to go. It was hot, humid and my head felt like it was on fire. I was out of touch with how I looked in comparison to my headshots. When I arrived at one location they didn't recognize me. I had to introduce myself to the person at the door and still they didn't seem to believe it was me.

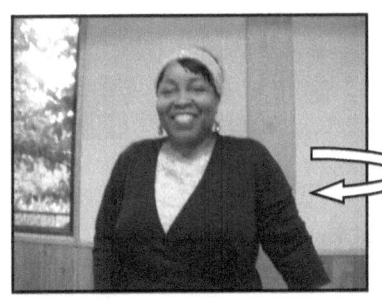

They were expecting the wavy-haired lovely in the previous photo but she arrived looking like this.

Wake up, fat girl.
(Photo taken Sept 2010)

At another location someone made the following comment about my recent CD cover photo. "Oh, this photo must have been taken when you were much younger." I was stunned for a moment. This photo was taken in 2006. I chose it for the CD cover because it captured my expression of joy. I had just put in a new weave on the day of the photo shoot so I just knew I was *fine*!

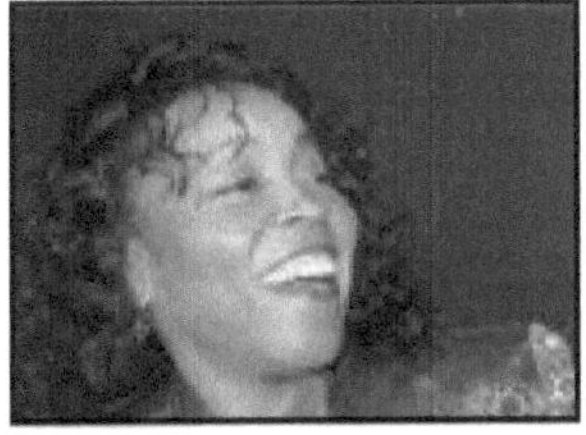

However, I never considered that my weight gain made me look so much older.

Rrrrrrring! Wake UP, Fat Girl!

A few weeks later, I met one of the organizers of the festival. It's amazing how a person can size you up with just one look. No matter how beautifully I sang, no matter what people said about my character, no matter how hard I worked, my appearance was the deal breaker. I knew it when I met him and received the two-second full body scan. Momentarily, his face said. "NO Way!" Then he broke into a grin, shook my hand and followed through with all the niceties. ("Nice-Nasties" as my mother would say).

I asked him. "Will I be invited to sing at the festival?
He said. "I'm not sure. We'll have to get back to you on that."

A few minutes later, right after I finished my song set, he announced from the stage that another singer was coming to be the headliner. People were asking. "Who?" He pumped her up so much that the Japanese people assumed she had to be a BIG STAR in America. The Americans present, including me, had never heard of this person. I knew then. I had been devalued, dismissed, not chosen. Why? Not because I lacked the talent or charisma, but because I was not attractive enough for their standards. I was too FAT. **GONG! WAKE UP, FAT GIRL!**

No one ever said it out loud. But I knew. I let a great moment in life get away because I'd developed a habit of satiating my emotions by overindulging in food. When I was tired, I would eat. When I was depressed I would eat. When I was lonely, I would eat. When I was frustrated, I would eat. When I was disappointed, I would eat. When I was happy I would eat. To celebrate, I would eat. Of course when I was hungry, I would eat.

Eating is only an appropriate response to hunger. I had no alternative outlet for my emotions and feelings. It was always food. Just like an addict, I'd medicate with food. Some choose shopping. Some choose smoking, exercise, sex, drugs, or alcohol. I chose food.

Suddenly my eyes were open to the way people responded to me. My Japanese friends were polite, but seemed very concerned for my health. When I had to walk or ride my bike, they would ask over and over. "Are you ok?" Apparently they noticed how hard I was breathing and how difficult it seemed for me physically. I was totally out of touch with my body.

My apartment in Japan is on the fourth floor. There is no elevator. When I first moved in lugging groceries or just my body up and down the stairs, my heart would race like it was coming out of my chest. Anyone going up the stairs with me would pass me and have to wait for me to catch my breath and finally meet them at the top.

A Japanese friend helped me take my clothes to the laundry center one day. Most Japanese people don't use a machine to dry their clothes. Instead they hang them on the balcony to dry in the sun. So, after the clothes were clean we had to bring them back up to the fourth floor…wet and of course much heavier.

When we got to the bottom of the stairs I was ready to take one end of the bag while she held the other to get the load up the stairs. She quickly threw the laundry bag of wet clothes over her shoulder and ran up the stairs with it. A few minutes later she was waiting for me at my front door. Yes, waiting for me to haul my out of breath, tired, fat, carcass up to meet her.

I was thankful for her help but very embarrassed. After she left, I realized how out of shape I really was. I was thinking. "This is not the person I want people to see when they look at me. People are treating me like a fragile old fat lady. I'm not old and I'm not fragile either. It was a rude awakening, but I finally woke up. Uuuuugh! I am FAT.

CONFESSION TWO

Living in a fantasy world.

I saw a commercial once where a woman was looking at herself in a full length mirror. Her body was a very nice healthy weight. The size most women aspire to be. No fat, no cellulite, nice curves, and very beautiful. Next the camera angle changed revealing her reflection. In the mirror she is obese and grossly overweight. The camera pans back to the live woman as she actually was, grossly anorexic, like a skeleton. The person she sees in the mirror is always too fat, no matter how much weight she loses.

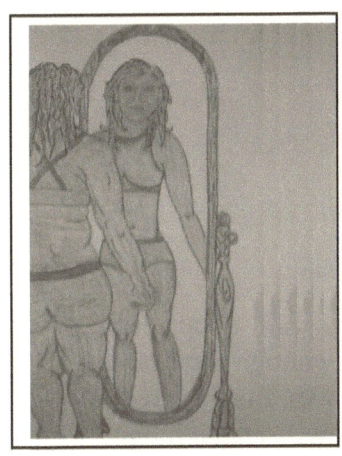

I think some obese women have the same problem but in reverse. For some obese women, no matter how much weight she gains, she still looks in the mirror and tells herself she is fine. This revelation is the inspiration for the drawing pictured here.

I watched a video blog of an obese woman who was starting a weight loss journey on the advice of her doctor. She was not taking it seriously at all. She made jokes as she removed fatty foods from her refrigerator and cupboards. She talked about the fact that her husband liked a woman with "a little meat on her bones". Though she was clearly at least 200 lbs overweight, she confessed that when she looks in the mirror, she doesn't see a serious problem.

For a long time I was only looking at myself from the waist up. I would focus on my face, my skin, my hair, and think to myself. "I'm o.k. I have great skin and teeth and look rather young." I compared myself to others who were also unhealthy, ignoring the weight problem that was staring me in the face everyday.

To maintain my obese body, I lied to myself, saying things like this.

"I have a large frame."
"I'm big boned."
"I'm just thick."
"I'm a BBW (Big Beautiful Woman)."

As Monique said in her film, *Phat Girls*.
"I'm not fat. I'm sexy succulent."

I told myself whatever would ease my guilt about eating another piece of fried chicken or piling enough food on my plate to feed a family of three. But I'm finally tired of promises on hold. I agree with my fellow Youtube blogger,

PlussizeKimonika, who says in her blogs. ***"I'm sick and tired of being FAT!"***

A friend gave me a full length mirror when I moved into my new apartment. For a few months I avoided the mirror because I couldn't connect with the woman I saw there. I haven't had a full length mirror in a long time.

Soon, I began looking at myself in the mirror. Not glancing… I mean really taking a long hard look. The blinders finally came off. I didn't like what I saw. I started asking myself some hard questions.

"Whatever happened to Beverly, the basketball guard, cheerleader, and softball player?"

"Where are those cute dimples and high cheekbones you used to show off when you smile?"

"When did it become ok to have a double chin and no collarbone?"

"Why do your wrists and ankles feel like you're wearing a sock around them?"

"What is all this hanging from the backs of your arms and around your waistline?"

"When did size 9-10 turn into size 20-22?"

Yes, I was living in a fantasy world where my weight didn't matter. At some point I had gained enough weight to become invisible. People no longer looked me in the eye. Maybe they were afraid their eyes would reveal what they were really thinking. "Wow! She's FAT!" On some level, I enjoyed being invisible. For a season I wasn't ready to manage all the things that come with physical attraction, especially from the opposite sex.

I still dream of falling in love and sharing my mature years with a nice gentleman. I dream of shopping in a regular section of the clothing store and finding things that fit… perfectly. I dream of going to the beach, wearing my swimsuit and actually getting in the water without embarrassment. I dream of performing onstage, knowing that I not only sound great but look fabulous! Afterward I want to enjoy the photos and video footage that back up that claim. That's the real me.

The time came for me to stop avoiding an issue that was obvious to everyone but me. People were not meeting Beverly. They were meeting that FAT unhealthy black woman with the beautiful voice. Michael Jackson said it best in his song, *Man in the Mirror*… "You gotta make that CHANGE today!"

CONFESSION THREE

Food memories and feeling loved.

When I was growing up I had two sets of god-parents. The Bradleys lived in Georgia. They were about the age of my grandparents...the sweetest people you'd ever want to know. My godmother, Mama Zadie, would stop her world at three o'clock everyday to cook dinner because my godfather, Daddy B. was on his way home.

Mama Zadie would go into her tiny old fashioned country kitchen everyday, no matter how hot or cold it was and throw down the best meal. She would cook fried chicken from scratch with all the seasoning, pork chops, collard greens with rutabagas, and so much more. She'd always add a little fatback or ham hocks to season the vegetables.

Mama Zadie would make hand rolled biscuits too! There was no recipe, just a lil' dis and a lil' dat. Mmmmm. Perfection! It was good ole' down home cookin'. Everyday she would thoughtfully set up a food tray at Daddy B's favorite easy chair, positioned in front of the television, so he could watch the Atlanta Braves during dinner.

When Daddy B arrived home from work at five thirty, he walked through the front door and began praising her as the smell of food wafted through the house. “Oooooh somethin’ really smells good in here. I know we ‘bout ta have somethin’ good today!” He would wash up and sit in that comfortable chair in anticipation. I watched him many days as he enjoyed his meal.

In the midst of telling off the referee in the Braves games, he never neglected to sandwich in some praise for Mama Zadie. “Oh, honey, you really put your foot in it today! This is the best meal you ever cooked.” He’d say. Her face would light up to receive this praise and the next day she would try to out do herself again.

Watching them taught me that food is a way to show your love and to receive love. I really believe that there’s nothing wrong with that understanding. However, people were less concerned about nutrition and weight issues back then. Our lives were naturally more physical and much of what we ate was quickly burned off. When I was a child back in the 1960’s we had to play outside until the sun was going down. We were not allowed to laze around the house watching T.V. We had no video games. We were not allowed to talk on the phone. So, we played kick ball, stick ball, rode our bikes or walked around the neighborhood.

Mama Zadie and Daddy B have both passed on now, but they will always have a warm place in my heart. That good home cooking experience gave me a feeling of being loved and nurtured.

My other godparents lived in Florida. They were about the age of my natural parents. They had four children. I made the fifth child so they had a full house. Mrs. Mary was a mother to me. We had the same complexion and were both chubby so people would mistake me for one of her natural children. Folks would ask her. "Mary, when did you have this child?" She would laugh and never answer the question.

Neighbors loved to come to my godmothers' house to eat. They would hang out for hours hoping they'd be around when she cooked. They would ask. "Whut you cookin' today, Mary?" Sometimes they would bring food over for her to cook because she could really *throw down*! (Translation: She was an awesome cook…restaurant worthy).

My godmother was an obese woman. She weighed over three hundred pounds, maybe more. She would cook and serve it lovingly. Everyone loved her because she was a big bundle of love.

Everything she cooked seemed to be fried or full of fat. I remember her delicious fried chicken, pork chops, burgers, fish, or shrimp. She made the best macaroni and cheese on the planet! It was sooooo good you would hurt yourself eating extra helpings until none was left.

We lived just off the bay where the shrimp boats would dock and sort their catch for the day. The docks were our front yard. Crabs, fresh from the shrimp boats were the only food that was boiled. I don't know what was in the crab boil, but it was *sho' nuff good* as the old folks would say down south.

Sunday was a special day because she would make a pancake breakfast for us kids: 2 pancakes, 2 sausage, 2 strips of bacon, and scrambled eggs with cheese. This was no Velveeta… but that guhvment (government) cheese. Some of y'all remember that big ole hard block of cheese the government used to give away to low income people back in sixties.

The pancakes were not palm-sized IHOP pancakes. They were the size of the bottom of the skillet….bigger than the size of my face. She always put a little bit of cornmeal in it. So they were heavy too. Oh yeah, I almost forgot the grits. We ate filling, high calorie foods. She saw to it that we left the table full. Don't get me wrong. It was delicious. But let me remind you. I'm only 5' tall. That's a lot of food for a little person.

My godmother, Mrs. Mary had lots of health issues. She passed away due to complications from diabetes. A few years later my god sister, one of her twin daughters, passed away from diabetes in her forties. A few years later, my godfather, her husband, also died as a diabetic.

My natural father died many years prior from… guess what… diabetes. Recently, I learned that my god sister, the surviving twin is also diabetic. So what can I learn from this? I'm sure my godmother was doing the best she could to feed us and give us good nutrition, but she didn't know it was not healthy. I've considered these childhood experiences very deeply in the past few months.

When someone cooks for you it is a very intimate and precious gift. I've learned to give and receive love through food over the years. It's true that when I come home and the house smells like good food; it gives me a really warm and loved feeling. It's a blessing when someone cooks for me.

Growing up like a foster child in other people's homes left me with many emotional scars. For most of my life I've struggled with feelings of abandonment, fear, unworthiness, and low self esteem. I learned to disconnect from people and things because people were not reliable and I never got to keep things of my own. The few things I enjoyed as a kid like toys and friends were either temporary or soon taken away.

The only joyful moments in my life were holidays like Thanksgiving, Christmas, July 4th, birthdays or anniversaries. These were celebrations with food as the central focus. All the church folks would gather as the mothers cooked their best dishes and laid them out buffet style. Everyone would eat till their hearts were content.

Of course everyone's belly was stuffed. There would be lots of laughter, ladies gossiping, men joking around, and us kids running around eating and playing. At church gatherings we were like one big happy family.

I fondly remember the Church picnics, fish frys, and bake sales. I don't ever want to lose these precious memories. It is a big part of who I am as a person. Enjoying the fellowship around home cooked food had become all important to my emotional well being. It was a big part of our culture when I was growing up in the South. The people I grew up with didn't have much. But, what they had, they shared freely.

My challenge now is to allow the emotion of love to come from the enjoyment of being with people so that the food can do what it was created for… to provide fuel for my body.

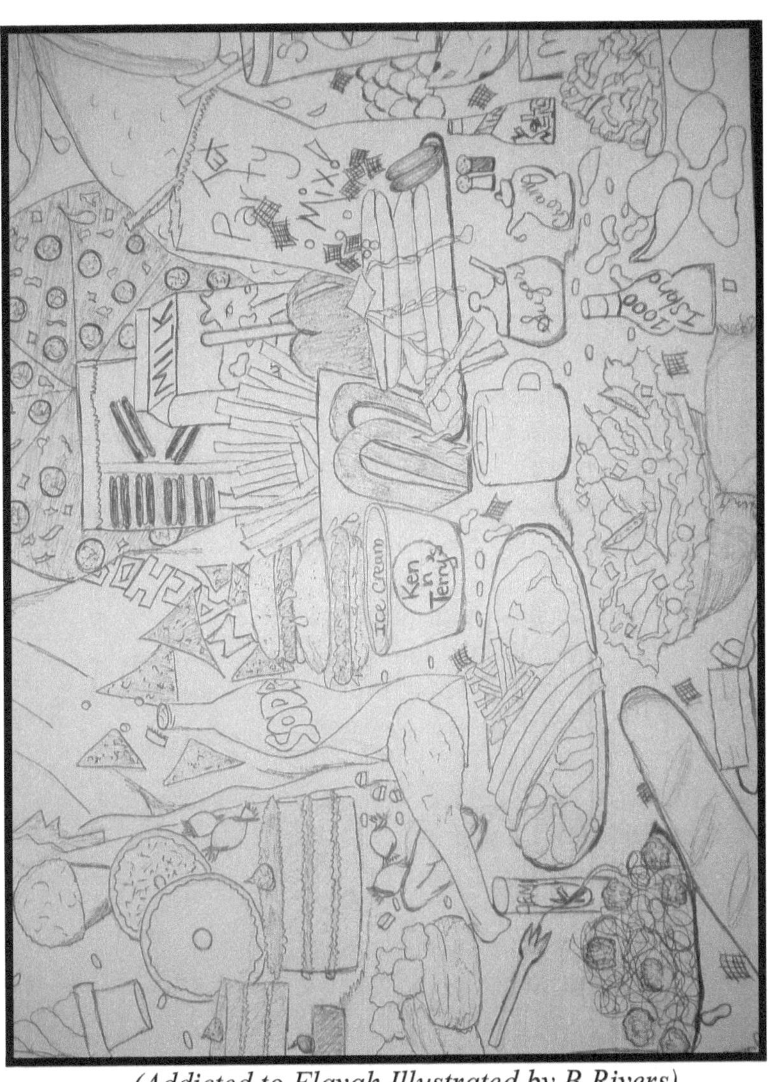

(Addicted to Flavah Illustrated by B.Rivers)

CONFESSION FOUR

In denial about my health

Sixteen years ago I was going through layered stresses of divorce, deaths in the family, job losses, and single parenting. I chose to medicate my emotions with food. The food brought back those good feeling of being loved when often I felt alone with all the challenges I was facing. For the first time I weighed in at 200 pounds and began experiencing various health issues.

I suffered from headaches, joint pain, nausea, and found it difficult to sleep. I would toss and turn at night and awake with one side of my body numb from poor circulation. I began worrying that maybe I was becoming diabetic.

Generally, I didn't feel well, so I went in for a physical. The doctor asked why I came in and I shared with him all my symptoms. He asked.

"Are you or anyone in your family diabetic?
"My father died from diabetes, but I'm not diabetic." I answered.
"What's going on in your life?" He asked.

I shared some highlights. He then ordered full blood work, and gave me a battery of other tests.

When the doctor came in to share the results I was sure the news would not be good. Instead he said. "You are not diabetic. Your blood pressure is good, actually a bit on the low side. Your cholesterol is ok. It could be better but it's not a serious problem. You are slightly anemic but that's not serious either. Then he closed the chart, looked into my face and said. "I'm surprised at these results. Most obese African Americans are also diabetic and have high blood pressure. So, this is good news! However, you are 100 pounds overweight. Do you realize that you should weigh 98- 110 pounds at your height?"

I just gave him a blank stare. His words felt like a shot to the heart. I was stuck on the word…OBESE. Did he just say OBESE?? Isn't that the word to describe grossly overweight people with medical problems? Isn't that the term for people who are about to die because they are too fat?"

Next, I rewound to the place where he said. "..You should weigh 110 pounds." He must be joking! I thought. I couldn't remember EVER weighing 110 pounds, not even as a child or a teenager. And I had never heard anyone use the word OBESE to describe me.

His voice interrupted my thoughts.
"You really need to lose weight or you will begin to have some serious health problems in the future. For now, I

suggest that you see a nutritionist to help you with choosing healthier foods for your diet."

I left the doctors office with mixed feelings. On the one hand, I was happy that I was not diabetic. On the other hand, over indulgence in food was the one vice that I could enjoy that was not illegal or immoral. I didn't want to think about how unhealthy it was.

A few days later, I met the nutritionist. She explained that she too was surprised by my physical exam test results. She asked.

"On a typical day, what do you eat?"

"Hmm…oh usually some chicken or fish…. Some kind of meat and vegetables at dinner time… I don't really remember." I responded.

Actually, I remembered, but was too embarrassed to confess that I could easily throw down three pieces of KFC, two biscuits, some mashed potatoes with gravy and of course a *diet* root beer. In the same day I could drive through McDonalds for lunch and grab a chicken sandwich or filet of fish sandwich, supersized fries, an apple pie and a strawberry shake. On top of all that, I'd eat a meal that I cooked at home that consisted of chicken or fish and some kind of vegetables.

The nutritionist told me to write down everything I ate and drank, including the time of day and quantity for one week.

Fifteen minutes after eating she wanted me to write down how I felt. During this first week she gave me instructions to keep a food journal without changing my eating habits at all. This exercise was eye opening. When I learned that a McDonald's shake had about half my daily calorie allowance, I completely cut them out of my diet.

Prior to my visit to the nutritionist, I did not realize how much food I consumed in a day. Most of my drinks were loaded with sugar. I drank very little plain water. Most of the foods were filled with salt, fat, sugar, and preservatives. Sometimes, I would eat and couldn't remember what or how much I ate. I would eat the food fast like someone was going to stop me or take it away from me. So, I consumed a lot of food before my brain had a chance to register that I was full. I ate until I was overstuffed and nauseous.

Often the food I was eating made me tired and sleepy. No matter how much I ate, I would be hungry again within an hour. Fifteen minutes after eating I would have a mild headache and my fingers and ankles were swollen.

One of my favorite binges was to pick up a 20 pieces of chicken tenders or four original recipe wings and eat it alone in my car so no one would see me eat. "Why?" You may ask. I had just eaten less than an hour before. I was not physically hungry, but emotionally hungry. Yeah, just like an addict I would hide my food. I craved salty crunchy snacks.

Another of my favorites was Chex Party Mix (cheese flavor). No matter what size bag I bought, I would top off the whole bag in one day, sometimes in one sitting. One handful of that stuff has about 200 calories.

When ever I cleaned out my car there would be at least five empty fast food bags and containers, crumbs from food that missed my mouth, stray French fries and snacks between the seats. When I wanted to eat… I wanted to eat now and not have to think about it, explain it, feel guilty about it, or apologize for it. I just wanted my food fix and that was it!

The nutritionist helped me learn that I am allergic to many preservatives found in processed foods. My body was struggling to digest the high fat, high sugar, and sometimes chemical ingredients. I was not eating enough fresh fruit, vegetables, and natural grains. I was not drinking enough water to flush the toxins out of my body. This explained why I was bloated, nauseated, constipated, suffering from headaches and found it difficult to sleep. The desire to do physical activities was only in my head. My body did not want to cooperate.

The nutritionist proceeded to tell me what I already knew. "You need to change your diet and lose some weight." She recommended a 1200 calorie diet that was mostly salads and lean meats. None of the feel good foods were on the list. You know them, ice cream,

donuts, cakes, desserts of any kind, fried foods, chips and dips, fast foods, or prepackaged foods. It just seemed like torture to me. Silently I protested, saying to myself. "If I can't at least enjoy eating… what else is there to enjoy?" I realize now that all along I've been dealing with a food addiction. I am a food addict! It's amazing that I never considered this until now, 20 years later.

The realization hit hard. Unlike other types of addictions, I can't just stop eating. I must control my eating. I must eat healthily and in proper balance with exercise. Somehow I had to figure out why I became an addict and correct what is going on inside. The thought of this was exhausting and a bit scary.

But now that I've awakened to the fact that I want my life back, I won't lie to myself anymore. I've asked myself. "How did I let this get so out of control?" I had to dig down deep and unpack some emotional problems, bad nutritional training, and a bad habit of using food to medicate depression. Now I'm committed to reclaiming my slim healthy body. I'm committed to being a good friend to you as well. There is a beautiful quote in the Bible that says.

"Faithful are the wounds of a friend; but the kisses of an enemy are deceitful." Proverbs 27:6 KJV"

I can't remember a friend or family member who was bold enough to give me the blunt and honest truth. Sadly, people only spoke with their reactions and not with loving words of correction. No one spoke up except my doctors.

Going forward in life, I want friends who will tell me the truth even when it hurts. Jesus modeled that type of friendship. When the woman at the well was lying to herself and living a messy life, Jesus called her out. That's true love and deep heartfelt friendship.

There have been people who stayed close to me for many years whom I thought were friends. In hindsight I can fully see that the relationship was one sided. Rather than seeing my greater good, these persons sought to take all they could and promote themselves.

So, my friend, if you weigh more than your ideal weight, according to your doctors assessment, don't kid yourself. Don't put your life off another day. Especially don't let someone else have to tell you you're fat! Look in the mirror and get real with yourself!

YOU NEED TO LOSE WEIGHT! NOW!

CONFESSION FIVE

Fat jokes are no longer funny.

One summer afternoon back in the 1970's, my husband, Wayne and I went to the San Jose Flea Market. It's a great place for an outing on a summer day when you don't have much money to spend. It's also a great place to people watch. All types of people are at the flea market, shopping, selling, or wandering around looking. We fell into the last category. Our favorite foods at the flea market were a chili dog and coke for him, corn dog and an orange soda for me. It was really hot that day…90 degrees easily.

We weaved in and out of little shops that sold fruits and vegetables, homemade tamales, or imported fabrics from India. A man covered from neck to wrist with glow in the dark necklaces, was walking around chanting "one dolla, two dolla". Even today I laugh out loud when I remember him.

Later we wandered through the rows and rows of people selling used items they harvested from their over stocked garages. This seemed to be my husband's favorite area since he spent most of his time looking at old tools and motorcycle parts for use in fixing his chopper.

Wayne started a long conversation about bikes with one of the sellers. Boring. So I left him to his new friend and walked across the isle to check out the costume jewelry displays. I looked through cheap necklaces,

bracelets and rings that would no doubt turn green after a little sweat hit them. As I turned to check on my husband, I spotted a very obese woman shaking her body left and right and pulling at her underwear through her dress. I thought, maybe she had an uncomfortable wedgie or something and was trying to work that out. I looked away thinking how embarrassing it must be especially with people staring.

A few moments later, I couldn't help myself. I had to look again. I turned just in time to see this massive woman part her legs and let her huge drawers drop to the ground. Then as if nothing happened, she stepped out of them and walked away with her male companion, leaving them sprawled out on the ground in full view. I'm not sure if the guy was her husband or boyfriend. Either way, he was shopping, totally oblivious to what just took place. By the way, he was super skinny. She was at least three times his size.

I abandoned my shopping and rushed over to interrupt my husband's chat. Grabbing his arm I asked. "Did you see that?" "Whut?" He grunted. Of course he was not even focused in that direction. I pointed to the large pile of fabric on the ground saying. "That!" He frowned and squinted a bit, cocking his head to one side then asked. "What's that?"… "Never mind."

OK. So by now you are either disgusted, or laughing your head off. It's just as well that my husband didn't witness that. I was shocked enough for the both of us.

This incident happened in the early 70's before my kids were born. Back then I weighed about 135lbs and wore a size 9/10 on top and size 11-12 on bottom. Yes, that's right. I've got those black girl child bearing hips. My husband loved it, though. My waist was small. I still remember my measurements… 36..28..42. I used to turn heads with those numbers, even though I still thought I was fat when compared to my sister who had a slim, dancer's body.

Now, let's fast forward to the 80's. I was hanging out with my two girls one afternoon and told them the story about the fat woman who dropped her drawers at the flea market. They thought I was making the story up. They were listening to a song that was very popular back then. "*Hey Fat Boy*" by Maximillan. All of a sudden I broke out singing new lyrics to the song …"Hey Fat girl, I think you dropped your drawz." We laughed so hard we were rolling on the floor crying.

Hey FAT Girl

Hey Fat girl, I think you dropped your drawz.
Hey Big girl, I really am appalled…na na na na na
Fat girl turn round and rounda
Her drawz drop to the grounda
She think nobody watchin'
All 'round her eyes are poppin'
Walk off like nothing change
Hey wait…is that a stain?

Hey Fat girl, I think you dropped your drawz
Hey Big girl, I really am appalled…na na na na na
Fat girl turn round and rounda
Her drawz drop to the grounda
Elastic stretched so wide
She need a bigger size
Lets run 'em up a pole
What country has three holes?

Uptown downtown all round da town
Fat girl don't care if her drawz fall down
Middle of the summer and her drawz fall down
Just can't believe I saw her drawz fall down.

Yeah, it was big laughs then, but a few years later it was not so funny anymore. When I saw that woman at the flea market, I never in a million years thought that I'd be obese. Overweight? Yes. I've been overweight according to rate charts all my life. But as a young woman I had slim firm abs, an athletic build, and was in excellent health. This flashback to the 70's and 80's caused me to recall and reflect on all the changes in my weight throughout my life.

During my senior year of high school, I played softball, basketball, and was a cheerleader. My cheerleading career lasted about two weeks. But, once I made the squad the thrill was gone. Jumping up and down, showing my underwear was not my bag. Sorry, I digressed a bit. Anyway… my point is…when I was young I took my health for granted.

At age 21, after my first pregnancy, I weighed in at 170 lbs. I remember feeling like a big bloated cow complete with milk jugs. Walking and breathing were such a chore near time for the delivery. After the birth of my beautiful little girl, I went into post partum depression. I tried to do a sit up and found out that my abs had turned into Jello. I lay on the floor and cried.

Eventually I lost 20 lbs, but my weight seemed to hover around 150lbs for the longest time. That last 15 lbs just never came off. My lifestyle then was very active with a husband, baby, job, and home to attend to. A few years

later when my second daughter was born, we lived in the country side. Life was quite sedentary there and I gained more weight. After her birth, I hovered around 165-170s. Over the years my weight gradually increased and my physical activity gradually decreased. In hindsight I can see that I needed to learn how to live a balanced life and give priority to maintaining my weight. There were days when housework was the only physical activity I did for days at a time. Soon my weight had gotten out of control.
I've bounced back and forth between 170 and 225 for about 15 years. I became the FAT GIRL in the lyrics I wrote years ago. It's certainly no laughing matter now.

You'll be happy to know that I inspect those drawers, (panties for all you delicate ladies) after every wash and discard them at the first sign of elasticity failure.

CONFESSION SIX

This is what depression feels like.

In the early 1990's, I was going through the worst trials of my life. I won't share the details, but suffice to say that I was living a nightmare. During this time, the emotional support I needed from family just wasn't there. I don't know what would have become of me without my church family.

For a few weeks I lived in the home of my Pastor, his wife and four kids while looking for an apartment. The stress and depression was so intense I remember feeling like I just wanted to step out of my body and go to another dimension. I can't say I wanted to commit suicide, but I truly wanted to make the emotional pain stop.

One morning I was ironing my slacks getting ready for work. My mind went blank. I was just standing there with the iron in my hand, staring at the wall. It was as if someone flipped the "off" switch and shut down all my body functions. A shadow walked past the open door to my room, backed up and called my name. I couldn't speak. A few moments later, another voice called my name. I couldn't respond. The voices sounded like muffled echoes down a long tunnel. I couldn't understand what they were saying. Someone gently took the iron from my hand.

The voices in the tunnel took turns speaking and seemed to come closer and closer. Finally my body rebooted. I looked away from the wall to see the Pastor's wife sitting beside me with her arm around me. The Pastor was ironing my slacks. They were both saying. "You're ok. It's going to be ok. Just keep going. Just keep trusting God. You'll get through this one day at a time." I'll never forget that moment. My spirit left my body.

Living in the home of others when I had very little income hindered me from indulging in my drug of choice without offending other people. Everyday I just wanted to scream but I couldn't. So, I began walking and praying out loud. I would walk until I was so tired all I could do was sleep. But, a short thirty minute walk became forty minutes, then one hour, and then.... Well let me share this story.

One day I went for a walk. I left the house around noon telling the Pastor's wife I would be right back. All I remember is walking, praying, and crying out to God about all the things that were going on in my life.

Suddenly I stopped walking, looked around and I didn't know where I was. It was kind of like that scene in the movie, *Forest Gump,* when he stops running and says. "I'm going home now." I turned around and started walking in the opposite direction hoping to see something familiar to find my way back to the house.

At some point I realized that my whole body hurt from head to toe. Every time I put my foot down to take a step, a pulse of pain would go through my body. My hip joints hurt and my legs felt like spaghetti noodles. All over my body I felt little popping sensations under my skin. I finally began to see familiar landmarks and made my way back to the house.

As I was nearing the driveway, I noticed a crowd of people standing on the front lawn. They were all church members, mostly deacons, the Pastor and his wife. They all looked at me with great relief. I was just about to ask what was going on when they quickly rushed to me making remarks like.

"Oh my God! Are you o.k?"
"Yeah, I'm fine. What's going on?" I replied.
They looked at each other in amazement. The pastor's wife asked.

"Where have you been? We were just about to call the police and split up to start looking for you." I was shocked.

"Why? Didn't I tell you I was going for a walk?" I asked. She responded.

"Do you know how long you've been gone? That was six hours ago and its almost dark now. We thought something happened to you."

I was stunned. I had no idea I had walked that long and I felt nothing until the last hour or so of my walk.

There is a nauseating feeling of anguish that tumbles inside my gut when I am depressed. I used to feed it with comfort foods that reminded me of happy childhood memories. Soon my belly would be full, and I couldn't feel the pain anymore. But during this time I couldn't medicate with food. Instead, I walked until the pain in my belly went away, but it was replaced with numbness. I couldn't feel anything. I had become so depressed it took six hours of walking for me to feel connected to my physical body again.

Depression is a very serious matter. Before this experience I did not understand how a person could get up enough nerve to kill themselves. I imagined that they would have to endure excruciating physical pain before they were actually dead. But this experience taught me that serious depression can cause a person's soul to disconnect from their body.

One becomes like a dead man walking. At this time one can feel no pain… just like when we are asleep… we are unconscious. There is numbness, a paused connection to life, and a constant unexplainable spiritual anguish that one wants to escape during times of deep depression.

I am not a psychologist. I'm just sharing my personal experience. For months I remember walking around in a daze functioning physically, but spiritually absent. My life was playing out before my eyes like a movie in which I felt I had no power to affect the outcome. This is a dangerous state of mind. For some they see suicide as the way out. But suicide is not the answer.

In the midst of the trauma, I learned that I enjoy walking. It relaxes me and lowers my appetite. During that time my goal was not to lose weight, but to my surprise, I lost three sizes without trying. Even after the day I got lost, I continued to walk, but for only one hour a day. I felt good. I started looking good too because suddenly men began to notice and comment. However, I did not enjoy the attraction at the time because I was dealing with the fall out of disastrous past relationships. The last thing I wanted was another man in my life.

When men began to flirt with me I felt overwhelmed and it triggered negative emotions that led to stress, that led to overeating, that led to lethargy, that led to less and less exercise, that led to weight gain….. again.

Years later, after slowly packing the weight back on, my car broke down and I had to learn how to get around using the light rail. I was finishing up my last year of Bible College. This time I *had* to walk. The station was about four blocks away from my home and about six blocks away from the campus. I lugged my books in a rolling flight bag while pounding the pavement for several months.

Determined to finish school on time I would not allow the absence of a car delay my graduation. I was so focused on school that sometimes I arrived home too tired to do anything but eat a cup of ramen noodles and go to sleep. I was not eating healthily but the weight was flying off. I lost about 35 lbs. Soon school was over. I bought a car and my activity level dropped significantly. I gained all the weight back.

Gain, lose, gain, lose…they call it the yo-yo syndrome. My weight was a reflection of my ever changing emotions. Nevertheless, walking was the beginning of healing for me.

In times of deep depression, it’s important to seek professional counseling. This is a time to cry out to God. This is a time to journal your feelings. This is a time for fasting and prayer. I did all of the above. By the grace of God, I’m still here to tell about it.

CONFESSION SEVEN

Generational addictive behaviors

My paternal grandfather was an alcoholic. He was an ex-military man who served in WWII. After giving his life to serve his country, the United States of America, he found himself unable to find work and provide for his family. It was a pivotal time in American history, years before Martin Luther King was old enough to begin peaceful protests about race relations.

My grandmother had to take up the slack. This meant working as a domestic in white people's homes for long hours with little pay. Often the pay was some second hand clothes, left over food and other things the lady of the house no longer wanted.

My father, also ex-military, was not an alcoholic, nor a smoker. However, the addictive behavior manifested itself in another way. Thankfully, he was a great people person and always managed to be working...often several jobs at once. As I consider his lifestyle, my father's drug of choice became sweet foods and sex.

He had entirely too many women in his life. It was a passion for him. Yet, it was demeaning and confusing for me, his daughter, to see his misbehavior and gross disrespect for women. It left me thinking that women could only expect to be used by men rather than receive love and respect. Sadly, I must admit that my father loved me, but he never modeled that love toward any

adult woman in his life so that I could have hope for a healthy relationship with a man in my future.

My father's addiction to sweet foods was also out of control. One of his girlfriends made him a three-layer chocolate cake for his birthday one year. By afternoon, he had eaten two thirds of the cake by himself! At this time he had already been diagnosed as diabetic. I was about 12 years old at the time and I remember saying to him.

"Daddy, the doctor told you not to eat so much sugar."
"You gotta die somehow. You might as well go happy!" He replied jokingly.

But of course, that was not funny to me. He was my only parent at the time. I didn't need to hear that he didn't care about living a healthy life and being around for me. My father had to take pills and insulin shots to control his sugar levels. As I mentioned before, he died in his early 60's from complications of diabetes. He refused to change his diet and live in balance.

As a teenager I came to live with my mother and step father. My mother has shared very little about her personal life as a young woman, so I'm unaware of any addictions in her life. However, I do know that my maternal grandfather was also an alcoholic.

So how does this all play out in my life? I am a third generation addict. There could be addicts further back but I don't know the history. My drug of choice is food.
Just like those before me, I overindulge knowing it's not healthy. Everyday I have to make positive affirmations and fight to overcome the urge to binge.

Many years ago a friend told me that she smoked to curb her appetite. She was very slim, so I got this dumb idea to try smoking. Armed with a pack of *Virginia Slims* cigarettes, I sat in my car at the park and smoked a whole pack of cigarettes one after another. Soon I was dizzy, coughing, nauseated, hoarse.... and still hungry. Afterward, I went to KFC, ate my favorite chicken meal, and gave up smoking.

I was not willing to exchange a thin body for an unhealthy, possibly cancerous one. Most of all I was not willing to sacrifice my singing voice to be thin. Singing is my joy! So I went home with a bad headache, a hoarse voice, and a tummy full of fast food. No more cigs for me. Great decision!

It's never a good idea to trade one bad habit for another. Anything in excess is potentially unhealthy. Addictions run in my family. Recognizing this helps me face the fact that it will take more than diet and exercise to permanently correct my problem. It's emotional, spiritual, and possibly hereditary. This will take time because I have many things to overcome. But, my eyes are wide open and I'm determined to end the generational cycle of addiction.

CONFESSION EIGHT

I'll never go back to FAT

The initial excitement of my arrival in Japan wore off at week four. Quickly I was faced with culture shock. The lifestyle here is very physical. Everywhere I go I walk or ride my bicycle to get from point A to point B. I don't drive a car at all. Instead I am constantly walking up and down the steps to the platforms at the train stations.

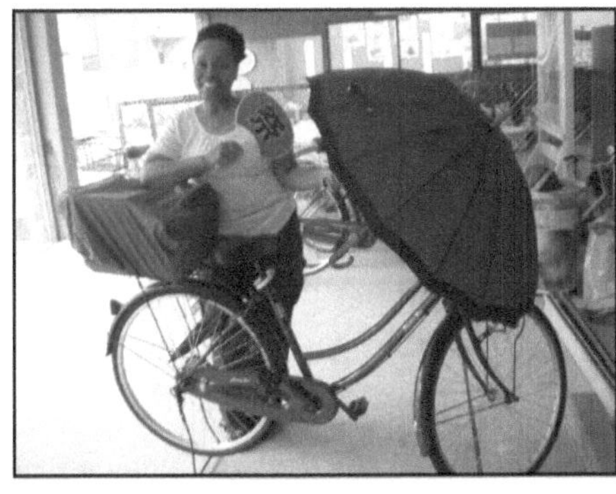

I live on the fourth floor of my apartment building. There is no elevator. So, I climb 72 steps up and down usually 2-3 times daily. Yes, I counted the steps because I want to remember all the components of my increased physical activity when this assignment is over. I will have to compensate for the calories I burn going up and down those steps everyday in order to maintain my weight loss.

At first, my diet was not much different than it was in America. I was still eating high fat, high carbohydrate foods and not many fruits and vegetables. Even so, I was slowly losing weight because of the increased activity.

The Japanese are known for their healthy eating habits and slim, petite bodies. In fact, Okinawans in southern Japan have been recorded as the longest living people on earth. But, times are changing. Fast food franchises are now all over Japan, all over the world for that matter. McDonalds, KFC, and Starbucks are in abundance here. These and other franchise restaurants make good money as many Japanese people become addicted to the foods high in fat, sugar, and preservatives. The ability to eat poorly still exists even in Japan where obesity is now becoming a concern.

My Japanese friends believe that American food consists only of hot dogs, hamburgers, French fries, corn dogs and pizza. It's unfortunate that we Americans have influenced others to abandon good health habits and join us in our struggle with heart disease, cancer, constipation, indigestion, poor nutrition, and obesity all for the enjoyment of good tasting food.

I realized months ago that the Japanese lifestyle presents the perfect environment for me to lose this weight for the last time. I set out to find ways to reach this goal. I bought a new scale and began weighing myself at the same time every morning.

I watched many weight loss journey videos online searching for tips and inspiration. I was especially inspired when I came across a blogger named ImpatientDieter. Her approach was fascinating because

she said that you have to reprogram your mind and do mirror work to be successful in keeping the weight off. Though I don't agree with many of her other methods, these two tips struck a chord with me. I agreed with her assessment that negative self talk and the wrong mindset will sabotage our efforts to get and stay slim.

Immediately I sought out positive spiritual and weight loss affirmations that I agreed with, created a playlist and began listening and repeating the confessions twice a day. Later I created my own list of affirmations from God's promises found in the Bible and began confessing those daily.
I also agreed with ImpatientDieter's discussion about mirror work. I soon began using the full length mirror my friend gave me. Everyday I look in the mirror and say the things to myself that I wished my mother and father had said to me as a young girl.

I Love you.
You are beautiful.
You are a royal princess
You are a blessing.
You can do anything you set you mind to.
Those dimples in your cheeks are cute.
What a nice outfit you're wearing.
You have great taste.
I expect wonderful thinks to happen for you.
I want the best for you

I also spend time in the mirror honestly evaluating myself, looking for ways to make positive changes.

Every confession you've read in this book is a memory that surfaced when I began to fast and pray for understanding about my weight problem. I needed to understand why I'm trapped in this cycle of weight loss and gain and why I let it get so out of control.

My problem is neither a medical issue nor a lack of knowledge regarding good nutrition. I fully understand that it's a simple math equation. If X=the number of calories needed to maintain my weight, and Y = daily calorie adjustment. Then X+Y will eventually result in weight gain. X-Y will eventually result in weight loss. Simply put, eat less, exercise more and the weight will melt away. The outcome is totally up to me.

The root of my problem has been my inability to manage stress and a lack of a strong desire to let go of my food addiction. Eating numbed my emotional pain and reminded me of times when I was happy and felt loved. I had become comfortable being FAT. It had become my fortress, the power used to repel relationships that I was not ready for. It gave me a sense of protection that I felt deprived of all my life. Protection that I should have received from loved ones when I was a child and young adult. My fat body had become a hiding place for my emotional brokenness.

As I considered all the memories and thoughts that came to me during my time of fasting and prayer, I realized that I don't need a hiding place, because the Lord my God is my protector, my healer, and the lifter of my head. He has never left nor forsaken me. Yet, I allowed fear and depression to overtake me. Instead of running to the healer and the lover of my soul, I ran to food and a fat covering for my comfort and protection.

At last I am outwardly living up to the person I see on the inside. Day by day I am becoming more and more like the woman God created me to be. I am coming to the end of that long dark tunnel I mentioned in Confession Six. I can see the bright sunlight and hear joyful voices laughing, living, and loving. I have the inner strength now to step out of my cocoon and be free to be me.

I decided to go on a liquid fast 3 days a week to pray and jump-start my weight loss. I removed all junk foods from my apartment and filled the refrigerator with fruit and vegetable juices. I also bought fresh green tea leaves, Chinese oolong tea, and instant miso soup. For three days my goal was to hydrate my body to flush out toxins. Daily I drank at least one full liter of clean fresh water and one full pot of green or oolong tea. I sipped tea all day long. When I had a taste for something sweet I would drink some fruit juice. When I had a taste for something salty, I would drink a bowl of miso soup.

As I fasted and prayed many memories came up in my dreams that helped me get some perspective. The first two days on the liquid fast were the most difficult. But, by day three, I felt light and was not hungry. I was surprised that even after three days with no solid food; I was still having full bowel movements. Yuuuuckkk!! (No this is not TMI –too much information… you need to know this!!) I was carrying around a belly full of waste that was just sitting there. I continued the three day liquid fast for about three weeks in a row.

A month later, my body felt clean, my skin looked clearer, and I lost about ten pounds. After each three-day liquid fast, I broke the fast by eating some salmon and some steamed green vegetables (green beans or spinach). The lessons learned from the nutritionist I consulted years ago were refreshed in my mind. So, the rest of the week, I logged my eating in a food journal and paid attention to how I was feeling after eating certain foods. The fasting and prayer time caused me to slow down and think before putting food and drinks into my body.

Six months into my journey, my weight loss was becoming noticeable. I had dropped two sizes in clothing. But I also noticed that when I had a day off I spent it in the apartment almost the entire day, creating my blogs, or working on the internet. Hours were spent sitting on my butt! An alarm went off in my head that shouted. "You can't sit on your butt all day long and

expect to lose weight permanently. You have to become more active… everyday!"

The excessive walking experience I shared in Confession Six taught me a very important lesson. The common denominator in losing weight without trying is movement. Several times I increased my exercise without thinking of it as exercise. This is an important key to maintaining my weight loss.

Armed with a better understanding, in January 2011 I made a commitment to start walking again. From that day on I began walking for one hour every day starting at 7:00am... rain or shine...even in the cold weather... no excuses! This time, however, I was not depressed, stressed out, or dealing with any negative circumstances or emotions.

Walking and talking with the Lord outside in the fresh morning air is relaxing and enjoyable. The combination of changes in diet and exercise caused the weight to fall off even more quickly. I began losing an average of about 1 lb a week.

Weeks later, I came across Dan McDonald, The LifeRegenerator. He was doing a video on green juicing. I listened to many of his discussions about how a raw food diet can heal, detoxify, and remove excess weight from your body. I decided to give it a try and purchased spinach, chard, celery, apples, ginger, and other ingredients to make my first green juice. I used a blender and squeezed the pulp through a cloth filter.

Later I decided to buy a juicer. Two days a week I would drink a quart of green juice for breakfast. During the rest of the day my meals consisted of fresh raw fruits and vegetables. My weight loss increased to 2lbs a week.
I was very excited to learn about the benefits of eating raw foods. I only ate raw foods about 80% of the time. Once a day I would eat a cooked meal that consisted of a small portion of fish or chicken, some cooked vegetables and a bowl of miso, corn soup, or egg drop soup. In Japan soups are thickened with corn starch rather than milk. Therefore it is much lower in calories. One cup has about 93 calories and 1gram of fat vs. 200 calories and 12 grams of fat when cream or whole milk is used.

Many years ago I eliminated pork and beef from my diet. After eating beef, I would feel tired and heavy like I swallowed a rock. It took days to digest red meat so I began eating it less and less until I no longer had a taste for it.

As for pork… well… I ate some pork at a retreat that looked like think sliced turkey. After putting it in my mouth I realized it was not turkey and it had a strange pungent odor. It made me nauseous. I've never desired pork since that day. When it is cooked in foods, I can smell that strange odor and my body says NO. So, I never buy pork or beef to cook at home. However, if a

friend serves it at her home, I try to be a good guest and eat what I am served so that I don't offend.

I enjoy eating like this because I can eat as much as I want without hunger or guilt. Whenever I miss the smell of food cooking in the kitchen, I buy some onions and garlic (mostly for the aroma), chicken or fish, my favorite vegetables, and one serving of rice, pasta, or bread. I cook a great meal that fills the house with that good home cooked food smell. Set the table, eat and enjoy!

Once a week I cook and sit down to enjoy as much as I want. I eat healthy foods so no guilt is necessary! I even eat out once a week. Often the menus in Japan give the calorie content of the dishes. This is a great help and I choose accordingly. This has become my general way of eating.

Something very interesting happened as the pounds were melting away. On March 10, 2011, Japan was hit with a massive earthquake and tsunami that left thousands of people dead, homeless, and completely devastated. Even though the people in the area where I live were not physically affected, the whole country was suffering from depression and the fear of the unknown. Even now, people are struggling to recover from the massive losses they have endured.

My teaching semester was coming to a close and it was time for me to go home to America for a visit. The students became concerned that I might not return to Japan, so every class planned a lunch or dinner outing to spend time with me before I left.

This was a most difficult time for maintaining my weight loss. For three weeks straight, I went out to eat about three times a week with heavy foods that I had not eaten for months. But I felt I couldn't say no, considering the situation. I was determined not to gain any weight back. So, on the day after having a heavy evening meal, I walked for 2 hours to burn off the excess calories. This was very challenging. I was doing great until I ate rice three days in a row, stepped on the scale and found that I had gained back four pounds! I was soooo upset!! It was freezing cold that morning and I went out for a two-hour long power walk.

When I got back I remembered The LifeRegenerator, Dan McDonald, and how he helped people to lose a pound a day by switching to raw foods. So, I challenged myself to eat only raw food for 9 days to see if I could lose 9 pounds and get back on track. Why 9 pounds? Well, I was 9 pounds behind the scheduled goal weight I had set for myself. Nine days later I had lost 9.2 pounds and I felt great! I also felt good about my accomplishment and my determination to keep the weight off in a healthy way.

About 80% of my diet continues to be raw fruits, vegetables and nuts. They keep my body clean, my breath fresh. Raw fruits and veggies are another key to maintaining my weight loss.

When I arrived in Japan on April 6th 2010, I weighed in at 225lbs. I lost ten pounds just from the change in lifestyle then began seriously focusing on losing weight. Today,

December 1, 2011, I weigh 165lbs. An additional 50 pounds is now gone forever because of the changes in diet and the increased exercise over the past year.

The ladies in my small group at church asked how much weight I had lost and why. My appearance changed so drastically, they became concerned about my health. I explained that I lost the weight on purpose by changing my diet and walking everyday for one hour.

One of the ladies had also been on a diet for quite some time but her weight loss was very slow. I invited her to walk with me in the mornings. She has been walking with me now for six month and has lost 25 lbs. Her energy level and stamina has increased and of course she is ecstatic about her accomplishments.

Gradually, other women joined us in the morning and the group has now grown to seven ladies. I never expected to influence so many people. We encourage each other to stay fit and take care of our health. The Japanese would say. “SUGOI!” (Cool!)

After going back to America and returning to Japan to continue my assignment, I decided to slow down and make sure that I am making permanent changes in my lifestyle and weight loss. I’ve lost weight many times before, but it all crept back and more. I am determined that the cycle will not repeat again.

In summary, I worked on my maintenance diet and exercise regimen from the beginning of this journey. In the past I would override my autopilot eating habits long enough to drop some weight, but as soon and I ended the diet, I slowly returned to my old eating habits and piled the weight back on. I never dealt with the root cause of the overeating or found any alternative solutions for maintaining the weight loss. This time, however, I am learning other ways to deal with my emotions, both good and bad.

Rather than celebrate with food all the time, I may buy my self something special, do a video blog, or call a friend and chat. In stressful situations I choose to go for a prayer walk or just take a nap to reset my day. I try to remember to eat when I am calm. I serve the food on plates and sit at the table rather than eat standing or while cooking. Now I eat, enjoy my food, feel satisfied and still maintain my weight.

I am no longer FAT but *FABULOUS!* That's what God created me to be, and that's what I am. I performed in a fundraising concert to benefit Japan earthquake and tsunami victims. I wanted to wear something red but could not find anything at the stores, so I designed and sewed this butterfly cape the night before the concert in April 2011. The concert was held during the celebration of Christ's resurrection. I felt like I was finally coming alive again too! I will never go back to being FAT.

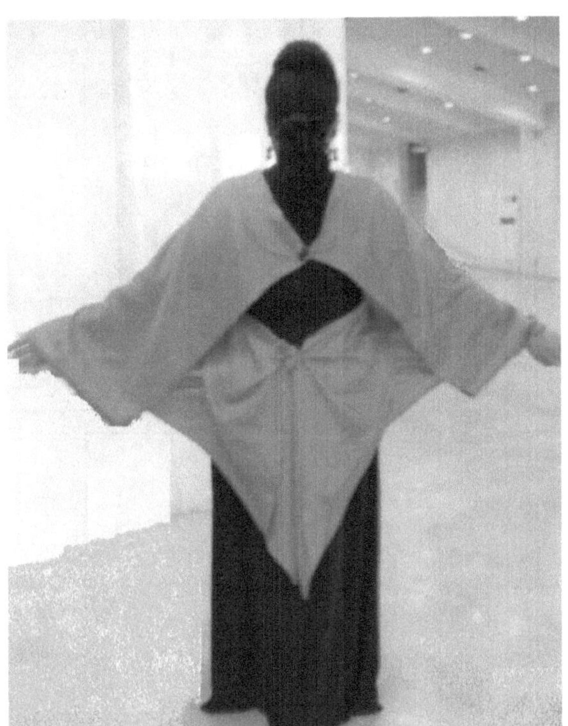

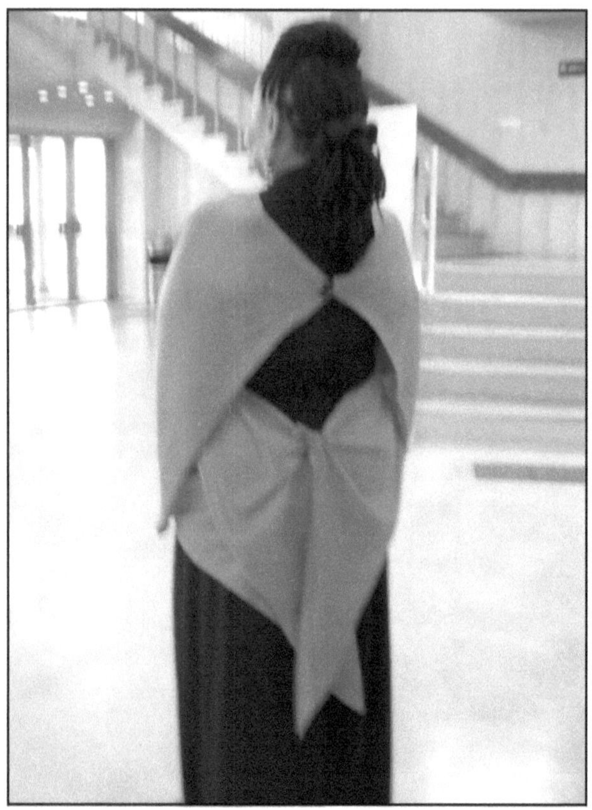

This cape reminds me of a story I wrote in 1994 entitled, *The Grub*. It is a fairytale about the metamorphosis of a very unlovely creature into a glorious one who spread her wings and sang to encourage others who were struggling along their way.

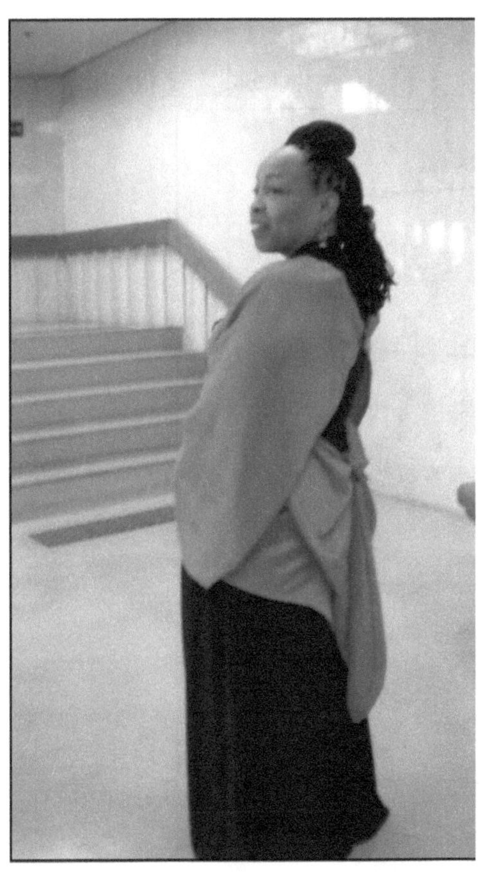

This journey has taught me some important lessons about myself. I was convinced that I had no sense of style. The truth is I have great style. Clothes I wore 50lbs ago were not tailored for a petite woman, so they fit like someone else's clothes and made me look even bigger. Now my clothes fit my body and my personality!

Ladies and gentlemen, meet . . .

Miss Beverly A. Rivers

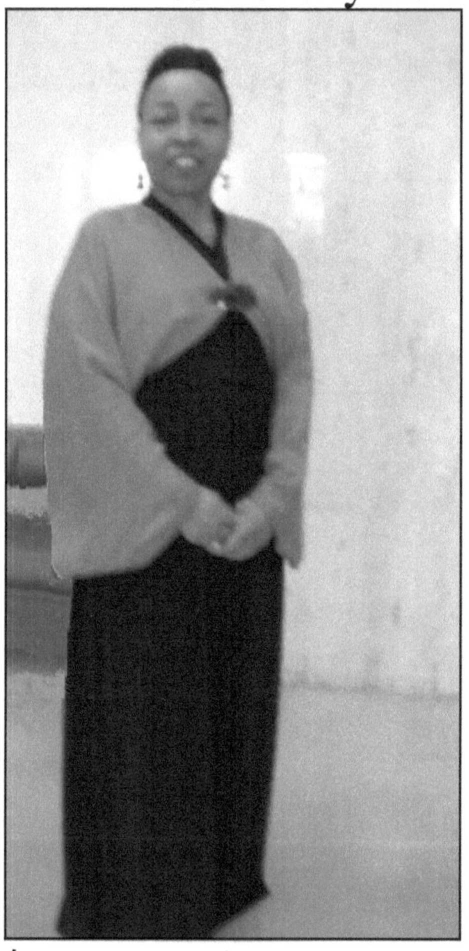

Princess Kizziemae

CONFESSION NINE

Ten ways my life has improved.

1. Increased Energy and Stamina

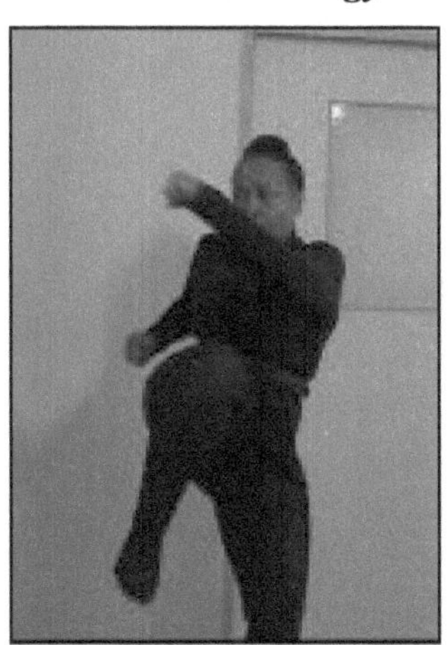

Sometimes I fly down the road riding my bike standing up. Halfway through my morning walk, I stop at a park and lead the ladies in 15 minutes of aerobic exercise. I can climb those 72 steps like a champ. I haven't had to carry laundry up the steps since that embarrassing day I mentioned early in this book. But, if needed, I could do it with no help. No sweat!

2. Fitting into Nicer Clothing Styles

I dropped four pant sizes and five jacket sizes. When I went home for a visit, my family was shocked to see how thin I am becoming. It was a good feeling to have people notice and tell me I was looking healthy and fit. I went from a size 20-22 down to a size 14 jeans (non-stretch levis) and a size 12 blazer. I could actually wear some stylish clothes and bought some cute pieces for my wardrobe. I also found some slim clothes in storage that I hadn't worn for years. Most of them were now too big. I was able to glean a few pieces that I can get a bit more wear out of. I realized that I have a great sense of style as a slim person, but as a plus size woman, few clothes looked attractive on me.

3. Younger Looking

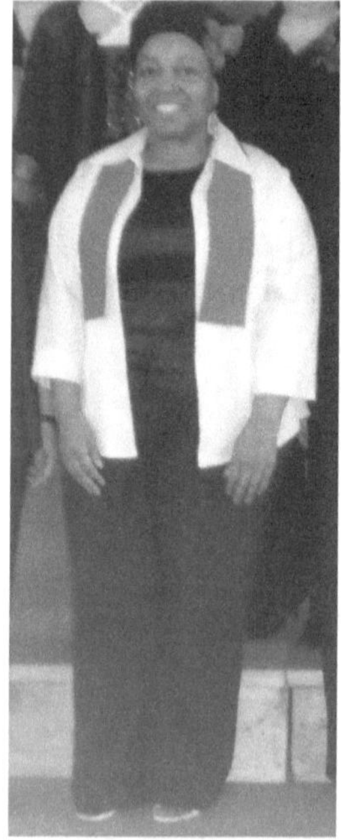

July 2010 – Before 225lbs

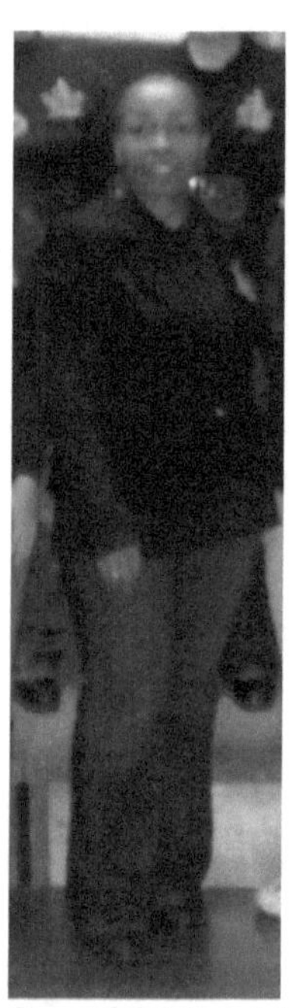

Sept 2011- After 165lbs

I've been told that I look younger and carry myself in a very youthful way. This is music to my ears because I don't consider myself old yet. I have so much to do before I retire to my rocking chair.

4. More Attractive to the Opposite Sex

Suddenly men notice me, open doors for me and seem to scramble to guide me up and down steps or into a car. I used to be uncomfortable with so much attention, but I'm enjoying in right now.

5. Eye Contact

I am no longer invisible. People seem to look me in the eye now whereas before, they would avoid eye contact. I'm not sure what to make of that.

6. Better Sleep

I sleep sooooo well now. I make it a point not to eat late at night anymore. After seven o'clock I usually just have fluids if I want something. I go to bed empty, sleep great, and wake up thinner!

7. More in touch with my body and what it needs.

I am getting to know when my body is dehydrated, needs protein, or needs to be detoxified. I can feel popping sensations when I'm burning fat. My skin itches when I've eaten too much as my body makes room to store the excess fat. For the first time in years, I actually hear my stomach growl signaling that I'm hungry. I smile when this happens because it means that I haven't been overeating.

8. I Like What I see in the Mirror.

I used to dread taking photos because I'd see them later and hate what I saw. But now, I'm happy to take and view my pictures with students and friends after concerts. I seem to get more photo opportunities too. Everyone wants a photo with their friend who is looking fabulous!

9. Inspiring others to become Healthier

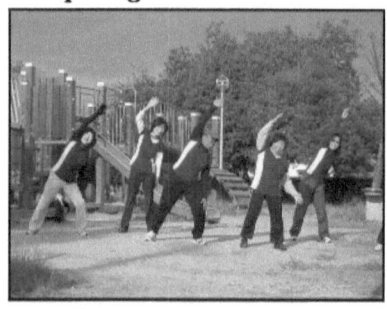

It is a great blessing that my success inspires others to become healthier. Some mornings I wake up and just don't want to go walking. In my mind I see all the ladies standing there waiting for me, so I get up and go. Once I'm out of the house… I feel energized and happy.

10. I Love Myself

I am finally becoming the person God says I am.

"I praise you because I am fearfully and wonderfully made. Your works are wonderful, I know that full well. My frame was not hidden from you when I was made in the secret place. When I was woven together in the depths of the earth, your eyes saw my unformed body. All the days ordained for me were written in your book before one of them came to be. How precious to me are your thoughts, O God!"(Holy Bible, Psalm 139:14-17 NIV)

CONFESSION TEN

Special dedication to a loved one who is morbidly obese.

This book is dedicated to someone I love very dearly who is morbidly obese. My dear one is at least 200 lbs overweight. I cried out to God about this because I have set a poor example that has contributed to this problem. I chose not to publish the identity of my dear one because my goal is to encourage not embarrass or offend. It has been my strong desire to correct this behavior so that my loved one can be healed body, soul, and spirit.

I am in a place of leadership in my family, the community, and now in Japan. For years I have shared my faith in God through song, testimony and teachings. All the while, I have used food as a comforter rather than trusting in Jesus Christ, my Savior and Lord.

"How can I lead the lost to Christ, but lose my way in this area of my life? This journey has convicted my heart. I must step up to the plate and lead by example. If I want my loved ones to be healthy and fit, I must prove that I believe what I preach. I must believe. "...***with God all things are possible."*** *(Matt 19:26)* ***"I can do all things through Christ who strengthens me."*** *(Phil: 4:13)*

For ten years I was a regular gospel performer at Higher Power, a 12-step ministry program of Central Peninsula Church in Foster City California. My band, Breakfree and I would go and share music that brought people to the altar in tears. Many of them were struggling with drug, alcohol, and sex addictions. It's ironic that the whole time I was there ministering to them, I never once thought of myself as an addict. Not until recently did I come to realize that I have more in common with them than I was willing to admit. I was drawn to that ministry because I needed it. I too was out of control.

Words without actions cannot fix this problem. I pray that my success in overcoming my food addictions will become contagious, not only for my loved ones but for all who read this book.

To my dear one:
I love you. Nothing can ever change that. I want you to live to see all your dreams come true. You're hiding a beautiful creation inside that fortress you carry around. This book is for you. With all your strength, press in and do what it takes to let the beauty inside break free. If you need me, I'm always here for you.

My closing thought is for everyone who reads this book. I would like to pray for your success and mine in the battle to overcome food addiction and live a healthy balanced life.

Metamorphosis Prayer *for our success*

Dear Lord Jesus, I come before you now thanking you for giving me everything I need to be successful in every area of my live. I believe that you exist and that you are a rewarder of those who diligently seek you.

My body was fearfully and wonderfully made by you. I was made in your image and after your likeness. Therefore, I am perfect, whole, and complete in you. I recognize that nothing is too difficult for you. Success is already given.

Please forgive me for using food as my comforter. You gave me your Holy Spirit to be my comforter, to teach me and show me all things. Help me to listen and obey your Spirit as you show me what to eat, when to eat and how to eat. Help me to obey when you tell me to pray. Give me the strength to abstain from overeating. Teach me healthy ways to deal with my emotions both good and bad.

Help me to spend more time in your presence. During my exercise times of walking or stretching, help me to hear your voice that calms me and guides me. Remind me that you have already given your life in payment for my sin including gluttony. Help me to forgive others so that I can receive forgiveness. Help me to forgive myself also. Give me the strength to let the past go and START OVER. In Jesus' name I pray. AMEN.

Princess Kizziemae's Daily Affirmations

I am fearfully and wonderfully made by God and I know that full well.

I am made in the image and likeness of God.

I am a royal princess, destined for greatness.

I am happy, whole, and complete in Jesus, Christ.

I love myself just as I am.

My body is the temple of the Holy Spirit, so I am careful to take good care of myself.

I pay close attention to what I put into my body.

I will not accept junk, leftovers, or garbage in any area of my life.

I deserve to be loved and cared for.

God gives me hope and a future. I receive it!

Jesus gave his life to take away my guilt and shame.

God has forgiven me, so I forgive myself.

I forgive everyone who has despitefully used, abused, and neglected me. I let them go.

I am strong in the Lord and in the power of His might.

Jesus promised never to leave nor forsake me so I am never alone.

Jesus promised that anything I ask for in His name, God the Father will do it.

All good things come to me at God's appointed time by His wisdom and knowledge.

I asked for healthy, loving relationships and I have them.

I asked for a slim, fit, and healthy body and I have it.

I asked for financial blessings and they are mine.

I asked for vision and purpose in my life and I have it.

I asked for my loved ones to be trim and healthy and it is so in Jesus' name.

I eat what I need to satisfy hunger then I stop.

I enjoy exercising everyday to stay calm and trim.

The Holy Spirit is my comforter. Food is my fuel.

I drink lots of water and tea all day long to stay hydrated.

Today I am excited about life!

Today something amazing is going to happen!

Today I eat lots of fresh fruits and vegetables and thank God for them.

Today my eating habits are being conformed to God's plan for me.

Today Godly love comes into my life and I embrace it.

I begin this day with thankfulness, joy and expectation!

I end this day with thankfulness, rest, and relaxation!

I am losing weight right now!

Today I am blessed and highly favored by God and people.

Today, God's mercies are new.

Today I START OVER!

Appendix

Resources
For Your Health Journey

Body, Mind, and Spirit

SELF EVALUATION QUESTIONNAIRE

Here are some questions I asked myself at the beginning of my journey. If you are joining me in this makeover and weight loss journey, take some time and answer these questions. Be honest and open with yourself. No one needs to see your answers. Give yourself at least one whole day to think about the questions and write down your answers. Take as much time as you need. Remember this is not a race, but a journey to the new you.

1. Close your eyes and think back to a day when you felt the most beautiful. Where were you? Who were you with? How old were you. How did you feel? What were you wearing? What color was it? Visualize yourself happy, healthy, and enjoying life. Describe it in the fullest detail as if you are making a diary entry.

2. Now, stand in front of a full length mirror. (If you don't own one, don't go any further until you get one. If money is an issue, you can probably find a cheap one at your local thrift store.) What are you wearing? Are you wearing this because you like it or because it fits? How do these clothes make you look? Old? Fat? Bigger? Thinner? Sloppy? Attractive? Describe an outfit you would buy if your size was not a factor.

3. Now, stand NAKED in front of the full length mirror. Get a good look at your body from all angles. Bend, stretch, squat, lift your legs and arms, and turn to see yourself fully. For a moment try to look at your reflection as if you are looking through a window at someone else. How do you describe the person you see? Have you known someone else in your past or present that looks like this? What do (did) you think of that person? Do you like what you see? Write ten sentences that describe the person you see in the mirror.

4. How do you describe the most excellent version of yourself? Pretend you are auditioning for a job where appearance is highly regarded or vitally important. (i.e. flight attendant, model, performer, public speaker, etc) Write a description of yourself as you would like others to see you. Use descriptions that are attainable for you even if they are not true right now. Be reasonable and realistic. Here's an example:

I am a, petite, African American woman, 5', weighing 135lbs. I am physically fit, youthful both in appearance and personality. Most people mistake me for 5 to ten years younger than my actual age ....etc.

5. Have the people around you met the real you? How do people treat you, look at you, and respond to you? Are you happy with that? Are you happy looking and feeling the way you do right now?

6. Can you remember what you ate for your last two meals? How often do you eat alone? How often do you eat in your car? How often do you eat standing up? When was the last time you heard your stomach growl signaling that you are hungry? Do you eat when tired, depressed, lonely, celebrating, and heartbroken? Are you a food addict?

7. Are you ready to change you life for ever? On a scale of 1-10, how committed are you? _______

List three behaviors you will work on over the next 30 days to begin your journey. Focus on changing one habit at a time. Work on it faithfully every day for at least 10 days or until it becomes a habit. For example: Habit Change 1: I will drink 1 liter of fresh clean water everyday for the next ten days.

Habit Change 1

____

____

Habit Change 2

____

____

Habit Change 3

____

____

KIZZIE'S SEVEN STEPS TO BETTER HEALTH

How I Lost 50 lbs and plan to keep it off.

Many who read this book have 100, 150, 200 pounds to lose. Fifty pounds may seem like a small accomplishment. I disagree. I truly believe that if you can lose 50 pounds while healing your emotions, dumping some baggage, and renewing your mind, you have set the stage for long term success.

I got serious and bought a scale. Every morning I weigh myself after elimination and before eating or drinking anything. I am confident that the second half of my journey will be so much easier. As I step on the scale I evaluate how my eating and exercise on the previous day effected my weigh in.

"A journey of 1000 miles begins with one step."
Lao-Tzu, a Chinese Philosopher

I encourage you to take one step, right now!

1. I CLEARED MY HEAD

Old tapes and memories had to come up and out. I separated myself from mentally stressful situation for a season and focused on my own needs. I reprogrammed my mind with truth from the word of God, the Bible. I spent time focusing on what I want from life. I took time daily to be thankful, dream and visualize my goals

2. I CLEARED MY CUPBOARDS

I removed everything from my house that would be a temptation for binging. That included salty snacks, fast foods, and sugary drinks. I replaced these with fresh fruits, fruit juices, fresh vegetables, soup bullion, instant low calorie soups, WATER, soy milk, and green tea.

When I was hungry, I had no choice but to reach for a piece of fruit, have a salad, or better yet, drink some water or tea.

A recent grocery shopping haul looked like this:
1 bag of apples
1 bag of oranges
2 large Japanese pears (so delicious)
2 bags of shredded cabbage mix for salads
2 bags of chopped mixed vegetables for making soup
(cabbage, sprouts, carrots, soy beans)
2 1 quart containers of soup broth
1 quart of soy milk
Roasted sesame salad dressing
Vinaigrette salad dressing

2 bundles of raw spinach
2 large onions
4 raw cucumbers
1 oz container of pickled radish
1 lb of chicken wings
(fatty yes! But I only eat them occasionally)
1lb of skinless chicken breasts
1 package of tofu
2 2oz pkg of water packed salmon

This was groceries for about one week. The apples and oranges may last for about 10 days. I eat out about twice a week. But when I do, I am choosy about what I put in my body. It must be fresh, rich in nutrition, look and smell good, and in harmony with my weight loss and maintenance goals.

3. I CLEANED MY COLON

For my first thirty days, I juice fasted for three days a week then ate sensibly for the remainder of the week. I broke the fast with dark green vegetables like spinach or green beans and some broiled salmon. Every remaining day of the week, I paid close attention to what I was eating.

Later in my journey I was introduced to green juicing. (See the appendix for a web link for a great green juice recipe) Green juicing is a great way to detox and kick start your weight loss.

4. I BEGAN WALKING EVERYDAY

I realized early on that to be successful I must burn more calories and be more physically active. I started by walking for 20-30 minutes a day and gradually increased to 1-2 hours. In general, I walked until I felt my body burning fat, then I turned around and walked home. I actually enjoy walking alone so that I can use the time to pray, meditate, and recite my positive confessions. However, sometimes it's difficult to be motivated to go alone. My walking partners help keep me accountable.

5. I STARTED DRINKING LOTS OF FLUIDS

After reviewing my food diary, I noticed that I was not drinking enough water or liquids in general. I was only having one bowel movement a day when I should have at least three. Lots of fluid is needed to flush out the waste I am burning off. So I began drinking one full pot of green tea daily and one full quart of fresh clean water.
I love coffee. However, coffee is a natural diuretic. Be sure to add another cup of water to chase the coffee and rehydrate your body.

6. I CUT OUT PROCESSED FOODS ONE BY ONE

As I became more in touch with how my body reacted to foods, I began to eliminate some. I ate less and less processed foods, fast food, and sweets. I cut out red meats (pork and beef) altogether. The only time I eat these is when it can't be avoided. (dinner guest, eat out with friends, etc)

Instead I began eating more and more raw fruits and vegetables, nuts, and soy products (milk, tofu, soy beans). For protein I chose chicken, fish, tofu, and nuts.

7. I MADE MYSELF TOP PRIORITY

I looked in the mirror everyday and told myself.
"I'm going to take care of you. You are hiding someone beautiful inside and its time for the world to meet her."

FOOD DIARY

When I began this journey I remembered my consultations with the nutritionist years ago. The food diary was a great way to evaluate what I was putting into my body and how it made me feel. I did this exercise again for about two weeks earlier this year. When I looked it over, I considered the content of foods that caused me to have a negative reaction within 15 minutes after eating.

I suggest that you try this too. Be sure to include quantities and as much detail as you can. You may want to make copies of the form below and fill it out daily for at least one month. Highlight the foods that are making you sick and sluggish. Try cutting back or eliminating those foods first. For me, the first thing to go was red meat. Later it was fast foods.

No one has to see this diary but you. So, be honest with your logging. If you ate 4 pieces of chicken, write it down. If you drank 2 glasses of wine, write it down. If you ate the whole cake, write it down. You will never accurately evaluate if you are not bluntly honest about where you are.

Also I must stress the importance of noting how you feel fifteen minutes after eating. When I realized that certain foods were giving me headaches, swelling and nausea I was motivated to cut them out of my diet.

Food Diary

Date: ____________________

Time	**Food Eaten**	**How do I Feel**

Ideal Weight Chart for Women

Height	Small Frame	Medium Frame	Large Frame
4'10"	102-111	109-121	118-131
4'11"	103-113	111-123	120-134
5'0"	104-115	113-126	122-137
5'1"	106-118	115-129	125-140
5'2"	108-121	118-132	128-143
5'3"	111-124	121-135	131-147
5'4"	114-127	124-138	134-151
5'5"	117-130	127-141	137-155
5'6"	120-133	130-144	140-159
5'7"	123-136	133-147	143-163
5'8"	126-139	136-150	146-167
5'9"	129-142	139-153	149-170
5'10"	132-145	142-156	152-173
5'11"	135-148	145-159	155-176
6'0"	138-151	148-162	158-179

(Based on Metropolitan Life Insurance Co. tables 1983)

Ideal Weight Chart for Men

Height	Small Frame	Medium Frame	Large Frame
5'2"	128-134	131-141	138-150
5'3"	130-136	133-143	140-153
5'4"	132-138	135-145	142-156
5'5"	134-140	137-148	144-160
5'6"	136-142	139-151	146-164
5'7"	138-145	142-154	149-168
5'8"	140-148	145-157	152-172
5'9"	142-151	148-160	155-176
5'10"	144-154	151-163	158-180
5'11"	146-157	154-166	161-184
6'0	149-160	157-170	164-188
6'1"	152-164	160-174	168-192
6'2"	155-168	164-178	172-197
6'3"	158-172	167-182	176-202
6'4"	162-176	171-187	181-207

(Based on Metropolitan Life Insurance Co. tables 1983)

RECIPES

Here are a few recipes. I eat as much raw fruits and veggies and I can but once a day I usually eat a cooked meal. A big part of the eating experience for me is to stimulate all my senses by seeing, touching, smelling, tasting, and even hearing the sizzling of the food cooking in the pan. It gives me joy, so sometime I cook just for me. I've learned to enjoy the eating experience by serving it on nice dishes at the table and sitting down to eat. I take a moment to thank God for his provision before I chow down!

Detox-Hydrate Salad

(No guilt, low calorie staple meal I ate whenever I got hungry. No matter what time of day. It's great as a breakfast to start the cleansing process.)

2-4 cups of raw cabbage/carrot salad mix
(cole slaw mix)

2 tbls of my favorite salad dressing
(roasted sesame seed) mix with 4 2bls of apple cider vinegar to stretch the dressing without adding calories.
2 raw cucumbers thinly sliced. Pile 'em on top

Still hungry??? Have another! No guilt!

Good Home Cooked Greens

(Sometimes I need to smell the food cooking in my house. So I enjoy making some greens with onions and garlic so the smell can waif through the house.)

1 bundle of raw spinach or other tender greens
1 fist sized white onion
2 cloves of raw garlic
2 fist-sized bell peppers
2 tbls soy sauce
2 tbls apple cider vinegar

I can easily eat this whole batch. I leave the table full and satisfied. If I'm craving some meat, I only eat half the batch of greens and add salmon or a chicken breast.

Broiled Mandarin Salmon
4oz pink salmon steak
1 cup of chopped onions, 1 clove garlic
1 mandarin orange
4 tbls apple cider vinegar
Seasonings to taste

Chop onions, garlic and place in a shallow dish. Add apple cider vinegar and seasonings. Place salmon steak in the mixture and allow it to marinate for a few minutes until cider is absorbed. Place salmon on foil in shallow pan and broil for a few minutes. until done. (time will vary based on thickness of the steak, but don't over cook) peel and wedge orange. Arrange the wedges on top of the steak and broil for three more minutes. Serve

KIZZIE'S AUTOPILOT EATING PLAN

Sample Daily Eating Plan – No calorie counting

I begin each day with a full glass of plain water, 1 cup of soy milk and a multivitamin supplement. I try to remember to let this be the first thing I put in my mouth.

I eat every two and a half to three hours so that I stay in control of what I eat.

Breakfast:

1-2 cups of shredded cabbage salad or other green vegetable salad. Enjoy 1-2 helpings as needed.

3-4 Tablespoons of my favorite salad dressing. Any kind I like with natural ingredients. Vinaigrettes are great. I stay away from artificially sweeteners because the chemical increases hunger. 1-2 helpings

2 fruits in their natural packaging, i.e. 1 medium apple, 1 medium orange. Peel and eat. 1-2 helpings

If very hungry add 1 boiled egg. Use non-caloric seasonings to taste.

Snack: 1 Fruit in natural package. (apple, orange, kiwi, pear, etc)
Drink: 2 glasses of water, non sweetened tea, coffee
Lunch:

1 bowl of soup broth, i.e. miso soup, beef bullion or chicken bullion soup. Some of these are quite salty so be sure to add lots of water. Add some chopped onions and chopped spinach for flavor and additional nutrition. Have 2-3 servings

1 cup of raw shredded cabbage and carrot salad mix. Top with ¼ cup of pickled radish, cucumbers, or 2 tbls of canned corn packed in water with no sugar added. Have 1-2 servings

If I'm very hungry top salad with 2.6oz of Pink Salmon or Tuna packed in water. (Chicken of the Sea pouches are 97%fat free and only 70 calories for all you counters)
1 serving only if needed.

Snack: Fresh fruit in natural packaging. 3 or 4 large dried plums or prunes. A handful of nuts.
(don't go crazy… nuts can slow your weight loss down)

Drinks: 2 glasses of water, non-sweetened tea, coffee in moderation but follow with water.

Dinner:

2 cups of stir fry vegetables

1 whole onion
2 oz tofu squares

Add 2 – 3oz of broiled or baked chicken or fish if you didn't have any at lunch time.

Add occasionally - 1 piece of toast, or ½ cup of whole grain rice, or ½ cup of whole grain pasta. (1-2 times weekly) These can also slow you weight loss progress. Watch the scale the day after you eat these to regulate yourself.

Dessert: Fresh fruit or small pastry under 200 calories or a latte with all the goodies in it. The choice depends on what I have a taste for that day.

Drinks: Water, water, water, at least one liter per day. Tea, tea, tea. Ooolong, green tea, herbal teas of all kind. I drink all day long.

So that's my simple daily eating plan. I eat chicken or fish when I'm feeling hungry and usually only once a day. For protein I eat boiled eggs, tofu, and nuts. All day long I'm drinking water, tea, or coffee. I stay hydrated. On weekends, I have one meal with no limitations at all. What ever my heart desires, I eat… including desert! Immediately the next day I go back to my normal daily auto pilot eating plan.

FOOD I HAD TO AVOID!

Bananas – For some reason, they just make me gain weight. There are naturally high in sugar content. I know there are a lot of banana diets out there, but they don't work for me.

Red meats – Beef and Pork. When I eat red meats, I feel weighed down and it takes a long time for them to break down in my intestines. So, days of walking around with meat in my body grosses me out now. Especially after my fasting and detox experience. I eat fish, chicken, and turkey they digest just fine for me.

White Bread, White Rice - These are highly processed foods and also seem to stay in my intestines a long time. Every time I ate bread or rice for two or more days a week, my weight loss would stall or I would begin to gain weight. Be careful and pay attention to your body and the scale.

Sweet Drinks – I stopped drinking soda pop years ago when I realized that the high sodium content was keeping me bloated. I buy unsweetened teas and coffees and add raw sugar or honey so that I can regulate it.

Animal Milk, Cheese, and Butter – I try to avoid these altogether because of the fat, lactose, and generally how they make me feel… weighed down. I use mostly soy milk, grated parmesan, and olive oil for cooking.

RELAXATION SUGGESTIONS

Alternatives to stress eating.

1. Go for a walk. Take deep breaths while looking and listening to the sights and sounds around your neighborhood. Pray and chat with God about how you're feeling.

2. Take a hot bubble bath with some good smelling oils and bath salts, Just soak and enjoy. Aaaaaah… Yes!

3. Turn on some soft music and do some slow yoga type stretches. Sometimes I turn on the music and make up my own interpretive dance to the song. If I'm angry, I put some fast music on and crazy dance like in the 80's movie "Flash Dance". I fight off the bad feelings and recite my affirmations to counteract the wrong messages I hear in my head.

4. Read the Bible or an inspirational book with positive messages on the topic you are stressed about. Most Bibles have a concordance or a reference index to help you find passages on any topic.

5. Recite your affirmation out loud to drown out bad thoughts or visions that come up.

Online Links for Inspiration

http://www.youtube.com/user/PrincessKizziemae
http://www.PrincessKizziemae.com

When you visit, please subscribe!!
Best Quote:
"Renew your mind and your body will follow."
Favorite Video: *Raw fruits and Veggies vs. Atkins*

http://www.youtube.com/user/liferegenerator

Best Quote: *"Can you dig it?"*
Favorite Video: *How to lose weight with raw food diet*

http://www.youtube.com/user/PlusSizeKimonica

Best Quote: "*I'm sick and tired of being FAT*"
Favorite Video:
10 Tips to avoid gaining weight during the holidays.

http://www.youtube.com/user/ImpatientDieter

Best Quote: "*This is the easy way show.*"
Favorite Video: *4 Steps to Success*

http://www.youtube.com/user/AsianSlimSecrets

Best Quote: *"Lose weight and stay slim for life."*

Fast Food Nutritional Fact Finder

McDonalds
http://nutrition.mcdonalds.com/getnutrition/nutritionfacts.pdf 16oz Strawberry Shake has 710 calories!!! Whuuut??

KFC, Kentucky Fried Chicken
http://www.kfc.com/nutrition/pdf/kfc_nutrition.pdf

Burger King
http://www.bk.com/cms/en/us/cms_out/digital_assets/files/pages/NutritionInformation.pdf

Pizza Hut
http://www.pizzahut.co.uk/restaurants/menus--deals/dietary-information.aspx The site is soooo pretty! So many beautiful pictures of the food before you get to the nutritional facts. Hmmmm.

http://www.pizzahut.ca/nutrition.htm
This one is more straight forward.

Krispy Kreme Donuts
http://krispykreme.com/nutri.pdf
one glazed donut ring has 200 calories! Wow!

Other Foods – Here's a great site.
http://www.caloriescount.org/calculator.html

Problem Cup

© 2010 By Beverly Rivers
Start Over CD release Hear it CDBABY.com

(Chorus)
Lord here is my problem cup and I pour it out to you.
I want you to fill me up
with you goodness, grace and kindness
Lord here is my problem cup and I pour it out to you.
I want you to fill me up.
Fill me up with you.

(Verse 1)
When I feel hard pressed on every side
And I think I'm about to lose my mind
When my problem cup is filled with worry, grief and pain.
I remember what you promised me
Then I lay my burdens at your feet
And I say fill my cup let it overflow with You.

(Verse 2)
When heartbreak brings tears to my eyes
And the words to pray are hard to find
When my tear pour out like heavy drops of falling rain.
I remember that you said. "Rejoice!"
So I lift my hands and use my voice saying
Father, fill my cup Let it overflow with You!
I want you to fill me. Fill me. Fill my cup with You!

Start Over

By Beverly Rivers © 2010
Start Over CD release Hear it at CDBABY.com

I can start over. I can start over. I can start over again!

He is the God who split the Red Sea
He's the God who said.
"March around the wall
and bring Jericho to its knees."
He is the God who wrote in the sand, saying.
"Who standing here can condemn you?
Not even one man!"

"START OVER!"

End Notes

So, my friend, you've reached the end of book one in Princess Kizziemae's makeover journey. I hope you are inspired. Please join me on this journey at:

Visit: http://www.PrincessKizziemae.com
Subscribers have access to my books and music at discounted prices.

Visit: http:/www.youtube.com/user/ PrincessKizziemae
This is my makeover channel where you'll find monthly updates, tips, and recipes. I subscribe to all who subscribe to my you tube account so that I may give and receive inspiration.

Visit: http://CDBaby.com
Start Over CD and other music releases can be heard and purchased online.

Friend me on Facebook. There are several Beverly Rivers' out there but only one me!

Follow me on twitter: @pkizzm

My next makeover blog book will be published after I reach my goal weight. I plan to weight 135lbs by August 1, 2012. Drop me a line and let me know how this book has impacted you.

www.ingramcontent.com/pod-product-compliance
Lightning Source LLC
Chambersburg PA
CBHW031236280526
45784CB00004B/1595

* 9 7 8 1 1 0 5 4 0 5 6 2 4 *